# RETURN TO LIFE

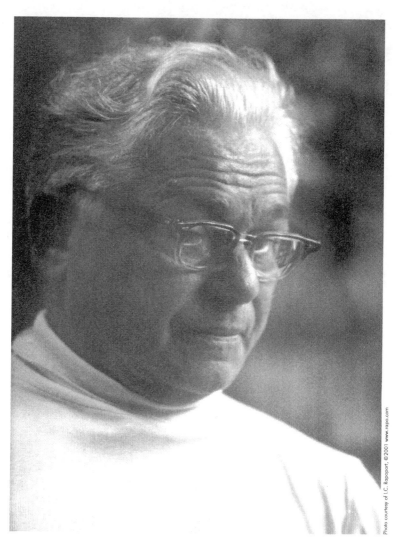

**Joseph H. Pilates**

# P I L A T E S'

## *Return to Life*
### Through Contrology

**by Joseph H. Pilates
and William John Miller**

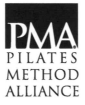

PILATES
METHOD
ALLIANCE

PILATES METHOD ALLIANCE, INC.
P.O. Box 370906
Miami, FL 33137-0906
866.573.4945
www.pilatesmethodalliance.org

Dedicated to "Clara"

# Contents

# Acknowledgment

The authors appreciate this opportunity to express thanks to all loyal friends and students for their sustained encouragement which cheered them onward in the preparation of this book. Special gratitude is acknowledged to Beatrice E. Rogers for most valuable assistance rendered, and to George Hoyningen-Huene for his unusual patience and exceptional professional skill in the production of the fine photography illustrating the technical text throughout RETURN TO LIFE.

Mortal perfection is achievable only through bodily perfection; and therefore the development of physique to high levels of strength and beauty, under control of the mind. This is the first requisite of human achievement. Also the maintenance of a superior standard of physical fitness is increasingly necessary to the maintenance of life and liberty in any complex civilization. It is supremely so in times of social strife. Therefore, the discovery and use of the most efficient programs of physical improvement are now vital to the very preservation of the race.

# Introduction

In my judgment, Contrology is an ideal system to transform the body into a perfect instrument of the will. It is kinesiologically proper, physiologically sound and, psychologically correct. I have personal knowledge of its success in effecting astonishing results, not only for normal adults but also for those suffering from sup-posedly incurable physical defects and organic deficiencies.

For twenty years I have studied professionally the leading sys-tems of body development proposed and used in schools, col-leges, private gymnasia, and other institutions, and have no hesitation in saying that the Pilates system is not merely 20 or 50 or 80 per cent more efficient, but must be several times as effective as any practicable combination of other systems.

To appreciate the truth of this statement the reader must himself have experimented with other systems, and then must have actu-ally used Contrology. For it develops not only the muscles of the body, suppleness of the limbs, and functioning of vital organs and endocrine glands; it also clarifies the mind and develops the will.

So it is with great pleasure that I endorse Joseph H. Pilates' work, and hope it will spread throughout our country, bring-ing increased physical fitness to all.

**Frederick Rand Rogers**
Former President
North American Physical Fitness Institute

# Foreword

For more than 40 years, Joseph and Clara Pilates worked to develop, perfect, and teach the exercise method they called "Contrology." While Joseph and Clara did not see widespread acceptance of the method during their lifetimes, today "Pilates" is one of the fastest growing exercise methods in the world. Joseph and Clara would have been very proud of the recognition their work now enjoys.

The Pilates Method Alliance is dedicated to the teachings of Joseph and Clara Pilates. Our goal is to define, protect and perpetuate the Pilates method, and to make the method understood and respected by those outside of the field, by establishing standards for certification and continuing education for Pilates teachers.

This reprint of Return to Life, complete with re-mastered photographs, is dedicated to Joseph and Clara Pilates, with gratitude.

**Pilates Method Alliance**

# The Basic Fundamentals Physical Education

**Civilization Impairs Physical Fitness**

Physical fitness is the first requisite of happiness. Our interpretation of physical fitness is the attainment and maintenance of a uniformly developed body with a sound mind fully capable of naturally, easily, and satisfactorily performing our many and varied daily tasks with spontaneous zest and pleasure. To achieve the highest accomplishments within the scope of our capabilities in all walks of life we must constantly strive to

# Of A Natural

acquire strong, healthy bodies and develop our minds to the limit of our ability. This very rapidly progressing world with its ever-increasing faster tempo of living demands that we be physically fit and alert in order that we may succeed in the unceasing race with keen competition which rewards the "go-getter" but bypasses the "no-getter." Physical fitness can neither be acquired by wishful thinking nor by outright purchase. However, it can be gained through performing the daily exercises conceived for this purpose by the founder of Contrology whose unique methods accomplish this desirable result by successfully counteracting the harmful inherent conditions associated with modern civilization.

In the Stone Age and onward man lived mostly outdoors with practically little shelter from the elements. He has not yet lived long enough indoors with protection against the elements to be able to successfully withstand the daily strains and stresses imposed upon him by our present mode of "fast" living. This explains why both you and I and all the rest of us are compelled in our own interest to give constant thought to the improvement of our bodies and to spend more time in acquiring and maintaining that all-important goal of physical fitness.

All in all, we do not give our bodies the care that our well-being deserves. True, we do stroll in the fresh air whenever our whimsical spirit moves us, or whenever necessity compels us to do so, with the result that on these occasions we do, in spite of ourselves, exercise our legs to this limited extent, accomplished, however, at the sacrifice of the rest of our body which after all is much more important to us from the viewpoint of our general health. Is it any wonder then that this haphazard and wholly inadequate body-building technique of the average person fails so miserably in the acquirement of physical fitness!

Admittedly, it is rather difficult to gain ideal physical fitness under the handicap of daily breathing the soot-saturated air of our crowded and noisy cities. On the other hand, we can more quickly realize this ambition if we are privileged to breathe the pure fresh air of the country and forests without the accompaniment of the traffic roar of the city which constantly tends to keep our nerves strung taut. Even those of us who work in the city and are fortunate enough to live in the country must counteract the unnatural physical fatigue and mental strain experienced in our daily activities. Telephones, automobiles, and economic pressure all combine to create physical letdown and mental stress so great that today practically no home is entirely free from sufferers of some form of nervous tension.

Because of the intense concentration demanded by our work and despite the real enjoyment our work may bring some of us we, nevertheless, gladly welcome any additional relief in the form of diversified and pleasant recreational activities, preferably outdoors, in our constant attempts to offset the effects of increasing cares and burdens so common today. To ease mental strain and relieve physical fatigue we must acquire a reserve stockpile of nervous energy in order that we may really be able to enjoy ourselves at night. Hobbies and all forms of play tend materially to renew our vitality with accompanying moral uplift. Play is not necessarily only confined to indulging in conventional games. Rather the term "play" as we use it here, embraces every possible form of PLEASURABLE LIVING. For example, simply spending a quiet and pleasant evening at home with our family chatting with congenial friends is, according to our interpretation, a form of play; that is, delightful, pleasant social entertainment as distinguished from our daily work. This finds us cheerful, contented, and relaxed.

However, many of us at the end of our daily work lack sufficient energy at night for recreation. How many of us simply spend the night routinely reading the evening newspaper? How many of us are entirely too exhausted to read, even occasionally, an interesting book, visit our friends, or see one of the latest motion pictures? When some of us occasionally spend a weekend away from our usual city haunts and environments, instead of receiving the immediate benefits of that desirable change in the way of complete revitalization (without fatigue) as the result of our experience outdoors in the bright sunshine, we are more often than not likely to find ourselves only recovering from the shock of our disappointment about the middle of the following week. Why? Because our previous mode of living and the consequent neglect of our bodies has not prepared us for reaping the beneficial results of this diversion. We lacked the necessary reserve energy to draw upon for this purpose and the fault lies only with us and not with nature as most of us like to think. All that any normal body should require is a change – from whatever it has previously been subjected to.

Accordingly, since we are living in this Modern Age we must of necessity devote more time and more thought to the important matter of acquiring physical fitness. This does not necessarily imply that we must devote ourselves only to the mere development of any particular pet set of muscles, but rather more rationally to the uniform development of our bodies as a whole-keeping all our organs as nearly as possible in their naturally normal condition so that we may not only be in a better position to earn our daily bread but also so that we may have sufficient vitality in reserve at night for the enjoyment of compensating pleasure and relaxation.

Perhaps with some feeling of doubt you ask, "How can I realize such a utopian condition? At night I am much too tired to go to a gymnasium." Or, "Isn't it too costly to enroll for a conditioning course in some good gymnasium or club?" RETURN TO LIFE fully explains how you can successfully achieve your worthy ambition to attain physical fitness right in your own home and at only nominal cost.

## Contrology Restores Physical Fitness

Contrology is complete coordination of body, mind, and spirit. Through Contrology you first purposefully acquire complete control of your own body and then through proper repetition of its exercises you gradually and progressively acquire that natural rhythm and coordination associated with all your subconscious activities. This true rhythm and control is observed both in domestic pets and wild animals – without known exceptions.

Contrology develops the body uniformly, corrects wrong postures, restores physical vitality, invigorates the mind, and elevates the spirit. In childhood, with rare exceptions, we all enjoy the benefits of natural and normal physical development. However, as we mature, we find ourselves living in bodies not always complimentary to our ego. Our bodies are slumped, our shoulders are stooped, our eyes are hollow, our muscles are flabby, and our vitality extremely lowered, if not vanished. This is but the natural result of not having uniformly developed all the muscles of our spine, trunk, arms, and legs in the course of pursuing our daily labors and office activities.

If you will faithfully perform your Contrology exercises regularly only four times a week for just three months as outlined in RETURN TO LIFE, you will find your body development approaching the ideal, accompanied by renewed mental vigor and spiritual enhancement. Contrology is designed to give you suppleness, natural grace, and skill that will be unmistakably reflected in the way you walk, in the way you play, and in the way you work. You will develop muscular power with corresponding endurance, ability to perform arduous duties, to play strenuous games, to walk, run or travel for long distances without undue body fatigue or mental strain. And this by no means is the end.

One of the major results of Contrology is gaining the mastery of your mind over the complete control of your body. How many beginners are amazed and chagrined (even trained athletes in the public eye) to discover how few (if any) Contrology exercises they are able to execute properly! Their previous failure to exercise regularly and properly, or their method of training, has not helped them. There is unmistakable evidence, too, that the functioning of the brain has correspondingly deteriorated. The brain itself is actually a sort of natural telephone switchboard exchange incorporated in our bodies as a means of communication through the sympathetic nervous system to all our muscles. Unfortunately, pure reason plays only a minor part in the lives of most of us. In practically every instance the daily acts we perform are governed by what we THINK we see, hear, or touch, without stopping first to analyze or think of the possible results of our actions, good or bad. As the result of habit or reflex action, we wink, dodge, and operate machines more or less automatically. IDEALLY, OUR MUSCLES SHOULD OBEY OUR WILL. REASONABLY, OUR WILL SHOULD NOT BE DOMINATED BY THE REFLEX ACTIONS OF OUR MUSCLES. When brain cells are developed, the mind too is developed. Teachers start with sense organs. Contrology begins with mind control over muscles.

By reawakening thousands and thousands of otherwise ordinarily dormant muscle cells, Contrology correspondingly reawakens thousands and thousands of dormant brain cells, thus activating new areas and stimulating further the functioning of the mind. No wonder then that so many persons express such great surprise following their initial experience with Contrology exercises caused by their realization of the resulting sensation of "uplift." For the first time in many years their minds have been truly awakened. Continued use of Contrology steadily increases the normal and natural supply of pure rich blood to flow to and circulate throughout the brain with corresponding stimulation to new brain areas previously dormant. More significantly, it actually develops more brain cells. G. Stanley Hall, the great American psychologist, observed: "The culture of muscles is brain-building."

## Guiding Principles Of Contrology

Contrology is not a fatiguing system of dull, boring, abhorred exercises repeated daily "ad nauseum." Neither does it demand your joining a gymnasium nor the purchasing of expensive apparatus. You may derive all the benefits of Contrology in your own home. The only unchanging rules you must conscientiously obey is that you must always faithfully and without deviation follow the instructions accompanying the exercises and always keep your mind wholly concentrated on the purpose of the exercises as you perform them. This is vitally important in order for you to gain the results sought, otherwise, there would be no valid reason for your interest in Contrology. Moreover, you must accept all collateral advice with equal fidelity. Remember that you are teaching yourself – right! The benefits of Contrology depend solely upon your performing the exercises exactly according to instructions – and not otherwise.

Remember, too, that "Rome was not built in a day," and that PATIENCE and PERSISTENCE are vital qualities in the ultimate successful accomplishment of any worthwhile endeavor. Practice your exercises diligently with the fixed and unalterable determination that you will permit nothing else to sway you from keeping faith with yourself. At times you may feel tempted to "take a night off." Don't succumb to this momentary weakness of indecision, or rather, wrong decision. Decide to remain true to yourself. Think of what would happen if the stokers firing the boilers of a giant oceanliner were to decide to "take a night off." You know the answer. If they were to repeat this action, you know the result. The human body, fortunately, can withstand more neglect, successfully, than can the complicated machinery of a modern steamship. However, that is no good reason why we should unnecessarily and unreasonably tax our bodies beyond bounds of endurance, especially since doing so results only in hurting ourselves. Schopenhauer, the philosopher, said: "To neglect one's body for any other advantage in life is the greatest of follies."

Make up your mind that you will perform your Contrology exercise ten minutes without fail. Amazingly enough, once you travel on this Contrology "Road to Health" you will subconsciously lengthen your trips on it from ten to twenty or more minutes before you even realize it. Why? The answer is simple: The exercises have stirred your sluggish circulation into action and to performing its duty more effectively in the matter of discharging through the bloodstream the accumulation of fatigue-products created by muscular and mental activities. Your brain clears and your will power functions.

## Bodily House-Cleaning With Blood Circulation

This is the equivalent of an "internal shower." As the spring freshets born of the heavy rains and vast masses of melting snows on mountains in the hinterlands cause rivers to swell and rush turbulently onward to the sea, so, too, will your blood flow with renewed vigor as the direct result of your faithfully performing the Contrology exercises. These exercises induce the heart to pump strong and steadily with the result that the bloodstream is forced to carry and discharge more and more of the accumulated debris created by fatigue. Contrology exercises drive the pure fresh blood to every muscle fibre of our bodies, particularly to the very important capillaries which ordinarily are rarely ever fully stimulated once we have reached adulthood. As a heavy rainstorm freshens the water of a sluggish or stagnant stream and whips it into immediate action, so Contrology exercises purify the blood in the bloodstream and whip it into instant action with the result that the organs of the body, including the important sweat glands, receive the benefit of clean fresh blood carried to them by the rejuvenated bloodstream. Observe the beneficial effects that Contrology exercises have on your heart action.

Contrology exercises guard against unnecessary pounding or throbbing of your heart. Study carefully the poses illustrated by the photographs and note that all the exercises are performed while you are in a sitting or reclining position. This is done to relieve your heart from undue strain as well as to take advantage of the more normal (original) position of the visceral organs of your body when in such positions. Contrary to exercises performed in an upright position, those performed while you are in a recumbent position do not aggravate any possible undetected organic weakness.

True heart control follows correct breathing which simultaneously reduces heart strain, purifies the blood, and develops the lungs. To breathe correctly you must completely exhale and inhale, always trying very hard to "squeeze" every atom of impure air from your lungs in much the same manner that you would wring every drop of water from a wet cloth. When you stand erect again, the lungs will automatically completely refill themselves with fresh air. This in turn supplies the bloodstream with vitally necessary life-giving oxygen. Also the complete exhalation and inhalation of air stimulates all muscles into greater activity. Soon the entire body is abundantly charged with fresh oxygen, a fuel which makes itself instantly known as the revitalized blood reaches the tips of your fingers and toes similarly as the heat generated by a good head of steam in your boiler and properly distributed by your radiators is felt in every room in your house.

Breathing is the first act of life, and the last. Our very life depends on it. Since we cannot live without breathing, it is tragically deplorable to contemplate the millions and millions who have never learned to master the art of correct breathing. One often wonders how so many millions continue to live as long as they do under this tremendous handicap to longevity. Lazy breathing converts the lungs, figuratively speaking, into a cemetery for the deposition of diseased, dying, and dead germs as well as supplying an ideal haven for the multiplication of other harmful germs. Therefore, above all, learn how to breathe correctly. "SQUEEZE" EVERY ATOM OF AIR FROM YOUR LUNGS UNTIL THEY ARE ALMOST AS FREE OF AIR AS IS A VACUUM. Stand erect again and observe how your lungs will automatically completely refill themselves with fresh air. The impact of so much oxygen upon your bloodstream may at first quite naturally and normally result in your experiencing a slight sensation of "lightheadedness," similar to the effect you might experience were you for the first time to find yourself actively engaged in the rarefied atmosphere high up in the mountains. However, after a few days this feeling will entirely disappear.

Whenever you read the word "rolling" in the exercises, be sure to hold your chin pressed tightly against your chest and, when you lie down or when you rise, "roll" and "unroll" your spine exactly in imitation of a wheel rolling forward and backward. Vertebra by vertebra try to "roll" and "unroll" as suggested. It is this very action of "rolling" and "unrolling" that cleanses your lungs so effectively by driving out the impure air and forcing in the pure air as you "roll" and "unroll." Indefatigably and conscientiously practice breathing until the art of correct breathing becomes habitual, automatic and subconscious, which accomplishment will result in the bloodstream receiving its full quota of oxygen and thus ward off undue fatigue.

Study carefully. Do not sacrifice knowledge to speed in building your solid exercise regime on the foundation of Contrology. Follow instructions exactly as indicated down to the very smallest detail. There IS a reason! Contrology is not a system of haphazard exercises designed to produce only bulging muscles. Just to the contrary, it was conceived and tested (for over forty-three years) with the idea of properly and scientifically exercising every muscle in your body in order to improve the circulation of the blood so that the bloodstream can and will carry more and better blood to feed every fibre and tissue of your body. Nor does Contrology err either by over-developing a few muscles at the expense of all others with resulting loss of grace and suppleness, or at a sacrifice of the heart or lungs. Rather, it was conceived to limber and stretch muscles and ligaments so that your body will be as supple as that of a cat and not muscular like that of the body of a brewery-truck horse, or the muscle-bound body of the professional weight-lifter you so much admire in the circus.

Concentrate on the correct movements EACH TIME YOU EXERCISE, lest you do them improperly and thus lose all the vital benefits of their value. Correctly executed and mastered to the point of subconscious reaction, these exercises will reflect grace and balance in your routine activities. Contrology exercises build a sturdy body and sound mind fitted to perform every daily task with ease and perfection as well as to provide tremendous reserve energy for sports, recreation, emergencies. Very interesting, but quite obvious when you stop to think of it, is the indisputable fact that no one modern activity employs all our muscles. The nearest approach to this ideal is found in all-round swimming and fancy diving. Walking, the only exercise over activity common to most of us, employs only a limited number of muscles. With repetition the art of walking becomes a subconscious habit, not infrequently a bad one, and only too often accompanied by poor posture--note our letter-carriers.

However, there is another important reason for consistently exercising all our muscles; namely, that each muscle may cooperatively and loyally aid in the uniform development of all our muscles. Developing minor muscles naturally help to strengthen major muscles. As small bricks are employed to build large buildings, so will the development of small muscles help develop large muscles. Therefore, when all your muscles are properly developed you will, as a matter of course, perform your work with minimum effort and maximum pleasure.

On a pleasant sunshiny morning, how we all naturally thrill in anticipation of accompanying congenial friends on a trip over modern highways to the country in a perfect-running automobile with a good driver at the wheel, knowing that his gradual acceleration and deceleration and his skillful negotiation of even sharp curves and abrupt turns are all accomplished so smoothly that we never give a conscious thought to his fine driving but rather concentrate on enjoying the passing scenery. How different, however, our reactions when taking a similar ride in a neglected car driven by a bad driver whose jerky starts, sudden stops, and dangerous turns not only upset our balance constantly but also rob us of the pleasure of the trip, especially after we realize that, luckily for us, he just missed "capsizing" the car although he did not succeed in avoiding dumping us into the ditch.

With the foregoing examples to guide us, we should wisely select as our pattern of life in this Modern Age that which excludes constant pushing, shoving, rushing, crowding, and wild scrambling all so characteristic of our day. This too fast pace is plainly reflected in our manner of standing, walking, sitting, eating, and even talking and results in our nerves "being on edge" from morning to night and actually depriving us of our needed sleep.

Constantly keep in mind the fact that you are not interested in merely developing bulging muscles but rather flexible ones. Bulging muscles hinder the attainment of flexibility because the over-developed muscles interfere with the proper development of the under-developed muscles. True flexibility can be achieved only when all muscles are uniformly developed. Normal muscles should function naturally in much the same manner as do the muscles of animals. For instance, at the very next opportunity, watch a cat as it lazily opens its eyes, slowly looks around, and gradually prepares to rise after a nap. First, it gradually rises on its hindquarters and then gradually lowers itself again, at the same time sprawling out on the floor, leisurely stretching its forepaws (with extended claws) and legs. Observe closely how all its back muscles actually ripple as it stretches and relaxes itself. Cats as well as other animals acquire this ideal rhythm of motion because they are constantly stretching and relaxing themselves, sharpening their claws, twisting, squirming, turning, climbing, wrestling, and fighting. Also observe, too, how cats sleep – utterly relaxed whether they happen to be lying on their back, side or belly. Contrology exercises emphasize the need for this constant stretching and relaxing.

Before proceeding, we must speak of the spinal column with which are associated practically all the major activities of our body. The spine is composed of 26 vertebrae. Each vertebra is separated from the other by intervertebral cartilage. This cartilage acts as a cushion to absorb the shock of sudden jars, reduces friction to a minimum, and gives the spine its characteristic flexibility, thus permitting it to function even more freely. The science of Contrology disproves that prevalent and all-too-trite saying, "You're only as old as you feel." The art of Contrology proves that the only real guide to your true age lies not in years or how you THINK you feel but as you ACTUALLY are as infallibly indicated by the degree of natural and normal flexibility enjoyed by your spine throughout life. If your spine is inflexibly stiff at 30, you are old; if it is completely flexible at 60, you are young.

Because of poor posture, practically 95 per cent of our population suffers from varying degrees of spinal curvature, not to mention more serious ailments. In a newly-born infant the back is flat because the spine is straight. Of course, we all know that this is exactly as intended by nature not only then but also throughout life. However, this ideal condition rarely obtains in adult life. When the spine curves, the entire body is thrown out of its natural alignment – off balance. Note daily the thousands of persons with round, stooped shoulders, and protruding abdomens. The back would be flat if the spine were kept as straight as a plumb line, and its flexibility would be comparable to that of the finest watch spring steel.

Fortunately, the spine lends itself quite readily to correction. Therefore, in the reclining exercises, be sure wherever indicated, to keep your back full length always pressed firmly against the mat or floor. When rising from the floor or lowering yourself to the floor, always do so with a "rolling" or "unrolling" motion exactly in imitation of a wheel, equipped with imaginary "vertebrae" rolling forward or backward. Vertebra by vertebra try to "roll" and "unroll." These "rolling" and "unrolling" movements tend to gradually but surely restore the spine to its normal at-birth position with its correspondingly increased flexibility. At the some time you are completely emptying and refilling your lungs to their full capacity. This admittedly requires persistence and earnest effort but – it is worth it!

It would be a grave error to assume that even Contrology exercises alone will remake a man or a woman into an entirely physically fit person. To understand this statement better, just remember that exercises as such with relation to physical fitness are somewhat similar to the relationship a grindstone or hone bears to an axe or razor. For example, how obvious is the answer to the foolish question as to which of two equally expert woodchoppers would cry "Timber" first, the one with a dull axe or saw, or the one who habitually sharpens his tools nightly in preparation for his work the next day. Correspondingly, proper diet and sufficient sleep must supplement our exercise in our quest for physical fitness. Another important factor in this connection is that of relaxation at stated fixed intervals throughout our workday wherever it is possible to do so, since this practice keeps us physically fit after we have obtained physical fitness. The man who uses intelligence with respect to his diet, his sleeping habits, and who exercises properly, is beyond any question of doubt taking the very best preventive medicines provided so freely and abundantly by nature.

By all means never fail to get all the sunshine and fresh air that you can. Remember too, that your body also "breathes" through the pores of your skin as well as through your mouth, nose, and lungs. Clean, open skin pores permit perspiration to uninterruptedly eliminate the poisons of your body. Moreover, unless you are really chilly, do not exercise in sweatshirts or even in lighter clothing. Whenever and wherever possible, wear "shorts" or sunsuits outdoors, and let the lifegiving ultraviolet rays reach and penetrate into every skin pore of your body. Do not fear the cold of winter. When you are outdoors wear rather loose-fitting clothes in preference to tight-fitting garments, not overlooking, of course, the importance of stout, comfortable shoes. Breathe properly, walk correctly, and swing along briskly. If you follow this sound advice you will find yourself feeling comfortable and invigorated.

The principal point to remember with regard to diet is to eat only enough food to restore the "fuel" consumed by the body and to keep enough of it on hand at all times to furnish the extra energy required on occasions beyond our normal needs and to meet unexpected emergencies. Merely eating to satisfy one's lust for good food is both foolish and dangerous to one's health. Such a person cannot ever be truly physically fit. No wonder! Youth and growing children quite naturally require a greater intake of food than do adults and the aged. The former are maturing; the latter have matured.

Not only the amount of food but also the kind is largely dependent upon one's occupation and sometimes, lack of it. Is it not reasonable to conclude that the sedentary indoor worker requires proportionately less food and of a different kind than the laborer who is engaged in hard manual toil outdoors? Heavy eating followed immediately by sitting, or even lying down awake or asleep, is comparable to overloading the firebox with coal and then closing the drafts of the furnace. The former instance is ideal for generating "poisons" that eventually find their way into your bloodstream. The latter instance is ideal if your aim is to maintain a smoldering fire without adequate heat instead of a bright, glowing fire to radiate its comforting warmth throughout your house. You have the choice in either case. Common sense dictates that you will make the right one. A man eating a heavy meal and indulging in vigorous activity will react thereto comparably to the way that a furnace with drafts open will react to a fire in a well-filled firebox. Accordingly, it is earnestly suggested that you guide your eating habits with all due respect to the required amount of food and kind you need to keep yourself physically fit, always as indicated by your occupation, or lack of it.

Often men who have been accustomed to work hard on a farm or play hard in school athletics or labor hard in a factory, continue eating the hearty meals they then ate even though now they are engaged only in sedentary indoor occupations where moderate meals are indicated. This practice is very unwise since it unnecessarily adds excess weight to their bodies, much of it in the form of undesirable fat which, if man were a hibernator, he could draw on in much the some manner that hibernating animals do in the winter when they draw against the stockpile of reserved energy with which the instinct of nature has provided them over the long period of their enforced inactivity and "sleep." Since man is not a hibernating creature, such excess of fat is a real detriment to him, imposing an unnecessarily heavy burden on his heart, liver, bladder and other vitally important organs of his digestive system. Still worse for him is the unnatural formation and accumulation of fat directly around the heart itself. The carrying of this extra poundage produces needless fatigue. Imagine yourself, for instance, carrying a well-filled traveling bag weighing 20 pounds. For one or two blocks, all goes comparatively well, but with each additional block it is carried the urge to rest is proportionately increased until at length the resulting fatigue compels you to do so. How relieved you feel after you have reached your final destination! You are doing exactly the very same thing when you persist in carrying 20 needless pounds of excess weight on your body only you are not so keenly aware of it because the weight is carried by the entire body instead of by your carrying arm alone as in the case of the bag. However, fatigue is created thereby in either case. Why not relieve yourself of this truly "excess baggage?"

Once acquired, it is, unfortunately, not so easy to rid yourself of excess weight. Nevertheless, it can be done! Consult your family physician for regular physical check-ups, and then follow his sound advice and instructions implicitly. Every adult over 40 years of age should not deny himself the benefits of a medical examination every three months. Once a year should suffice for younger persons unless some condition indicates to the contrary. Even in their case, consulting their physician twice a year would be wise. If this sound suggestion is followed, latent ailments can be discovered in their early developmental stage, and the "growth" of a long and perhaps serious illness may thus be "nipped in the bud."

If any particular part of your body is under-developed or shows an accumulation of excess fat, select Contrology exercises specifically designed to correct the respective conditions, repeating the exercises at stated intervals throughout the workday whenever it is possible to do so. However, be sure NEVER TO REPEAT THE SELECTED EXERCISE(S) MORE THAN THE PRESCRIBED NUMBER OF TIMES since more harm will result than good by your unwittingly or intentionally disregarding this most important advice and direction. Why? Because this infraction creates muscular fatigue-poison. There is really no need for tired muscles. Judicious selection of special Contrology exercises will accomplish more for your health and bodily condition, in conjunction with the foregoing advice, than all else combined.

Now let us consider the important question of good sleep at night. A quiet, cool, well-ventilated room is best. Do not use a soft mattress. "Firm but not soft" is a good rule to follow. Use the lightest possible bed coverings consistent with warmth. Do not use large bulky pillows (or as some do, two stacked pillows) – better still, use none at all.

Most important in the matter of enjoying good recuperative sleep are quiet, darkness, fresh air, and mental calm. Nervousness is usually aggravated by a lack of proper exercise, especially in the case of one with a troubled mind. The best alleviative for this condition is exercise. So if your sleep is disturbed, rise immediately and perform your exercises. It is far better to be tired from physical exertion than to be fatigued by the "poisons" generated by nervousness while lying awake. Particularly beneficial in this regard are the spinal "rolling" and "unrolling" massage exercises which relax the nerves and induce sound, restful sleep.

While conceding the fact that nowadays practically everyone of us routinely indulges in daily baths, experience has nevertheless taught us that only a small minority really achieve thorough cleanliness thereby, from our point of view. In our opinion, the correct technique to use in accomplishing this highly desirable result is to use only a good stiff brush (no handle) since this type of brush forces us to twist, squirm, and contort ourselves in every conceivable way in our attempts to reach every portion of our body which are otherwise comparatively easy to reach with a handle brush. The use of a good stiff brush as described stimulates circulation, thoroughly cleans OUT the pores of the skin, and removes dead skin too. The pores of your skin must "breathe" – they cannot do so unless they are kept open and freed from clogging. Your skin will soon respond most gratifyingly to this perhaps seemingly "Spartan-like" treatment and acquire in the process a new, fresh, glowing appearance, and develop a texture smooth and soft to the touch. So brush away merrily, and heartily too!

Finally, beginning with the introductory lesson, each succeeding exercise should be mastered before proceeding progressively with the following exercises. Make a close study of each exercise and do not attempt any other exercise until you first have mastered the current one and know its routine down to the last detail without any reference to the text. Be certain that you have your entire body under complete mental control.

## Results Of Contrology

Good posture can be successfully acquired only when the entire mechanism of the body is under perfect control. Graceful carriage follows as a matter of course. Just as a good smooth-running automobile engine is the result of proper parts correctly assembled so that it operates with a minimum consumption of gasoline and oil with comparatively little wear, so too is the proper functioning of your own body the direct result of the assembled Contrology exercises that produce a harmonious structure we term physical fitness reflecting itself in a coordinated and balanced tri-part unity of body, mind, and spirit. This in turn results in perfect posture when sitting, standing, or walking with the utilization of approximately only 25 per cent of your energy while the approximately remaining 75 per cent in the form of surplus energy reserve is "on call" to meet the needs of any possible emergency.

The art of correct walking consists principally and simply in a slight tilting forward of the proper standing posture, alternately placing one foot before the other with the weight of the body poised and balanced on the balls of the feet. Be careful not to lock your knees as doing so will jar the spine and interrupt the rhythmic walking motion.

Standing also is very important and should be practiced at all times until it is mastered. First, assume the correct posture, then when tired, shift the weight of the body from one side to the other while resting on the "idle" side. Do not push your hips out or lock your knees. Progress forward with a slightly swaying graceful motion comparable to the effect created by a gentle breeze blowing over a field of growing wheat ready for harvest, causing it to gracefully sway in "waves" from its roots to its tips. Never slouch, as doing so compresses the lungs, overcrowds other vital organs, rounds the back, and throws you off the balance created by poising the weight of your body on the balls of your feet.

If you will faithfully follow the instructions, beginning with the introductory lesson, you will without doubt acquire correct physical fitness with proper mental control. You will truly be building upon the solid foundation of Contrology which itself is built upon scientific principles so true, sound and unique that the science and art of Contrology will live forever. As you progress in your self-instruction, you never have anything to "unlearn." These exercises will actually become a part of your very self securely stored away forever in your subconscious mind. You who have learned correctly how to ride a bicycle, how to swim, or how to drive an automobile need never worry with respect to the possibility of your failing to use the right technique in these skills on all occasions because of the confidence born of the fact that you realize you received your instructions from the best available source and authority. So, too, the acquirement and practice of the art and science of Contrology will instill that confidence in you that will remain forever for future use as occasions therefor may indicate. Then it is simply only a question of "re-toning" the muscles that have in the meantime become "soft" as the result of disuse.

With body, mind, and spirit functioning perfectly as a coordinated whole, what else could reasonably be expected other than an active, alert, disciplined person? Moreover, such a body freed from nervous tension and over-fatigue is the ideal shelter provided by nature for housing a well-balanced mind that is always fully capable of successfully meeting all the complex problems of modern living. Personal problems are clearly thought out and calmly met.

The acquirement and enjoyment of physical well being, mental calm, and spiritual peace are priceless to their possessors if there be any such so fortunate living among us today. However, it is the ideal to strive for, and in our opinion, it is only through Contrology that this unique trinity of a balanced body, mind, and spirit can ever be attained. Self confidence follows. The ancient Athenians wisely adopted as their own the Roman motto: "Mens sana in corpore sano" (A sane mind in a sound body). And the Greeks as a people displayed even greater wisdom when they practiced what they preached and thus come nearest to achieving its actual accomplishment. Self-confidence, poise, consciousness of possessing the power to accomplish our desires, with renewed lively interest in life are the natural results of the practice of Contrology. Thus we achieve happiness, for is not real happiness truly born of the realization of worthwhile work well done, with the gratification of enjoying the other pleasures flowing from successful accomplishment with its compensating measure of "play" and resulting relaxation?

So in your very commendable pursuit of all that is implied in the trinity of godlike attributes that only Contrology can offer you, we bid you not goodbye but "au revoir" firmly linked with the sincere wish that your efforts will result in well-merited success chained to everlasting happiness for you and yours.

# The Exercises

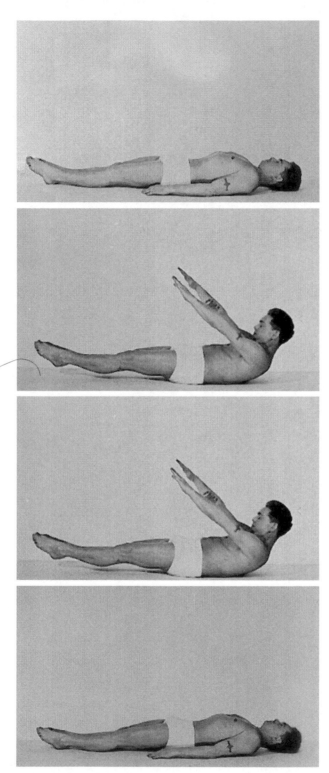

## The Hundred
Introductory Exercise

**Pose 1**   (a) Take position illustrated

(b) Lie flat with body resting on mat or floor

(c) Stretch arms (shoulder-wide, touching body, palms down) straight forward

(d) Stretch legs (close together, knees locked) straight forward

(e) Stretch toes (pointed) forward and downward

**Pose 2**   (a) INHALE SLOWLY

(b) Lift both feet about 2" above mat or floor

(c) Raise head with eyes focused on toes

(d) Raise both arms about 6" to 8" above thighs

**Pose 3**   (a) EXHALE SLOWLY

(b) Raise and lower both arms (tensed)

(c) From shoulders only

(d) Without touching body

(e) Within a radius of 6" to 8"

(f) Mentally counting 5 movements while

(g) EXHALING SLOWLY

(h) Alternating with 5 similar movements while

(i) INHALING SLOWLY

(j) Begin with only 20 movements and

(k) Gradually increase them in units of

(l) 5 additional movements each time until a

(m) Maximum of 100 movements is reached

(n) Never exceed 100 movements

**Pose 4**   (a) Relax completely

**REMARKS**   At first you probably will not be able to carry out instructions as illustrated in poses – this proves why these exercises and all succeeding ones will benefit you. However, with patience and perseverance you eventually should succeed in achieving the ideals as posed – with accompanying normal health.

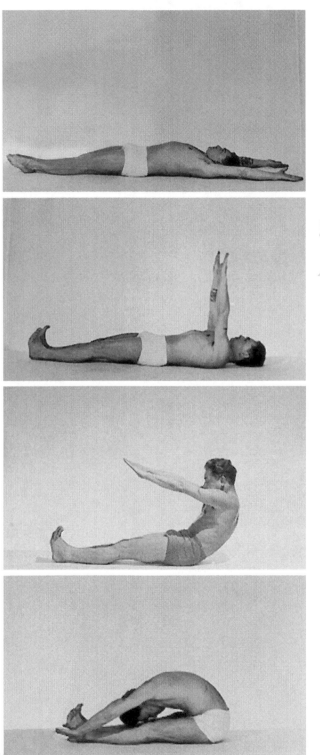

**Pose 1**  (a) Lie flat with entire body resting on mat or floor
       (b) Stretch arms (shoulder-wide, palms up) straight backward
       (c) Stretch legs (close together, knees locked) straight forward
       (d) Stretch toes (pointed) forward and downward

**Pose 2**  (a) Begin INHALING SLOWLY and bring arms (shoulder-wide)
           straight forward to upright right angle position and
       (b) Toes (pointed) upward

**Pose 3**  (a) While still INHALING SLOWLY
       (b) Bend head forward and downward until
       (c) Chin touches chest and then
       (d) Begin EXHALING SLOWLY and
       (e) Start "rolling" slowly upward and straight forward

**Pose 4**  (a) While EXHALING SLOWLY finish
       (b) "Rolling" forward until
       (c) Forehead touches legs and then
       (d) Begin INHALING SLOWLY while returning to Pose 3 and
           Poses 2 and 1

*NOTE*  Repeat the foregoing exercise three (3) times, trying with each repetition not only to stretch the entire body more and more but also to reach farther and farther straight forward as indicated.

*CAUTIONS*  Pose 1 – Entire spine must touch mat or floor. Tense body (do not bend arms or legs).
Pose 3 – Press both legs against mat or floor; if at first unsuccessful, placing cushion on your feet will materially help you.
Pose 4 – Legs must remain flat on mat or floor (knees locked). Palms must remain flat on mat or floor (arms stretched straight forward).

*REMARKS*  This exercise strengthens the abdominal muscles, and restores the spine to normal.

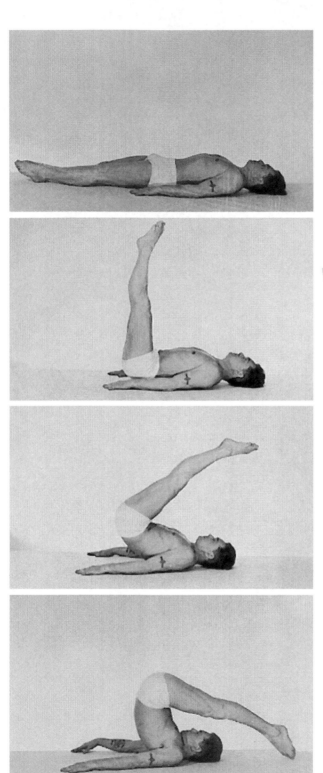

### The Roll-Over
### With Legs Spread
Both Ways

# The Roll-Over With Legs Spread

**Pose 1**    (a) Take position illustrated
             (b) Lie flat on mat or floor
             (c) Stretch arms (shoulder-wide, touching body, palms down)
                 straight forward
             (d) Stretch (close together, knees locked) straight forward
             (e) Stretch toes (pointed) forward and downward

**Pose 2**    (a) INHALE SLOWLY and
             (b) Begin raising legs upward and over until
             (c) Toes touch mat or floor
             (d) EXHALE SLOWLY and
             (e) Press arms firmly against mat or floor
             (f) (Spread legs as far apart as possible)

**Pose 3**    (a) INHALE SLOWLY and
             (b) Begin "rolling" slowly downward with
             (c) Both legs (tensed) straight (and spread as far apart as
                 possible)
             (d) Until spine touches mat or floor
             (e) EXHALE SLOWLY while
             (f) Returning to position illustrated in next pose below
             (g) With legs about 2" above mat or floor

*NOTE*    Repeat foregoing exercise five (5) times with legs close together at the
         start of first movement and five (5) times with legs spread apart as far as
         possible at the start of the second movement.

*CAUTIONS*    Pose 3 – Keep legs (tensed, knees locked) as for apart as possible.
                    Roll downward slowly from one vertebra to another.
            Pose 4 – Keep back and head firmly pressed to mat or floor.

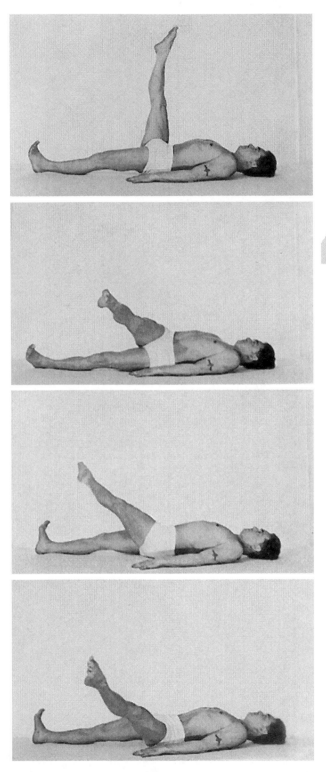

## The One Leg Circle
Both Ways

**Pose 1**   (a) Lie flat with entire body resting on mat or floor
        (b) Stretch arms (shoulder-wide, touching body, palms down) straight forward
        (c) Bring right leg to upright right angle position
        (d) Stretch toes (pointed) forward and downward
        (e) Left toes upward

**Pose 2**   (a) Begin EXHALING SLOWLY at start of downward motion with right leg while making a complete left-to-right circle (in the air) over the left thigh, then
        (b) Begin INHALING SLOWLY at start of upward motion with right leg in completing this circle
        (c) Begin EXHALING SLOWLY at start of downward motion with left leg while making a complete right-to-left circle (in the air) over the right thigh, then
        (d) Begin INHALING SLOWLY at start of upward motion with left leg in completing this circle

**Pose 3 and Pose 4**   (a) Begin INHALING SLOWLY at start of upward motion with left leg while making a complete right-to-left circle (in the air) over the right ankle, then
        (b) Begin EXHALING SLOWLY at start of downward motion with left leg in completing this circle
        (c) Begin INHALING SLOWLY at start of upward motion with right leg while making a complete left-to-right circle (in the air) over the left ankle, then
        (d) Begin EXHALING SLOWLY at start of downward motion with right leg in completing this circle.

**NOTE**   Repeat the foregoing exercise five (5) times with each leg.

**CAUTIONS**   Pose 1 – Toes must be pointed forward and downward (knee locked), right leg. Keep left leg (knee locked) flat on mat or floor with toes "pulled" upward and backward. Shoulders and head must always remain flat on mat or floor.
Pose 2 – Same as Pose 1 but note that right hip is raised.
Pose 4 – Same as Pose 2 but note that left hip is raised. "Swing" left and right legs as far as possible when making circles. Shoulders and head must always remain flat on mat or floor.

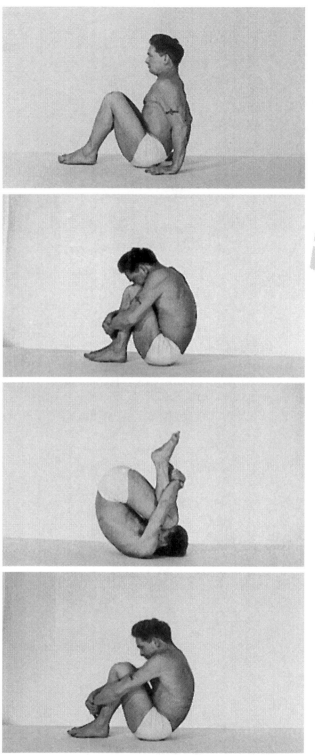

**Pose 1**    (a) Take position illustrated

**Pose 2**    (a) Grasp legs tightly with locked arms
             (b) Try to press thighs to chest
             (c) Bend head forward and downward with chin touching chest
             (d) Toes (pointed) forward and downward
             (e) INHALE SLOWLY
             (f) "Rock" backward to Pose 3 position

**Pose 3**    (a) EXHALE SLOWLY while
             (b) Returning to Pose 2 position

*NOTE*    Repeat the foregoing exercise six (6) times.

*CAUTIONS*    Pose 2 – Press chest in, round back, head down; keep feet off mat or floor.

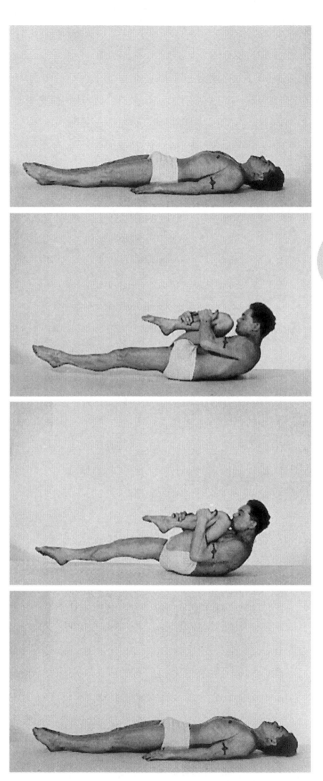

**Pose 1**    (a) Lie flat with entire body resting on mat or floor

**Pose 2**    (a) Bend head forward until
              (b) Chin touches chest, then while INHALING SLOWLY
              (c) Clasp hands and
              (d) "Pull" right leg as for as possible toward chest
              (e) Keep left leg stretched forward (knee locked)
              (f) Stretch toes (pointed) forward and downward with
              (g) Heel raised (about 2")

**Pose 3**    (a) While EXHALING SLOWLY
              (b) Clasp hands and
               (c) "Pull" left leg as far as possible toward chest
              (d) Keep right leg stretched forward (knee locked)
              (e) Stretch toes (pointed) forward and downward with
              (f) Heel raised (about 2")

**NOTE**    Repeat the foregoing exercise five (5) times with each leg.
(Later on the number of repetitions may be gradually and progressively safely increased to twelve (12) times with each leg.)

**CAUTIONS**    Pose 2 – Chin must touch chest. You must see your toes. Heels must be raised (about 2").

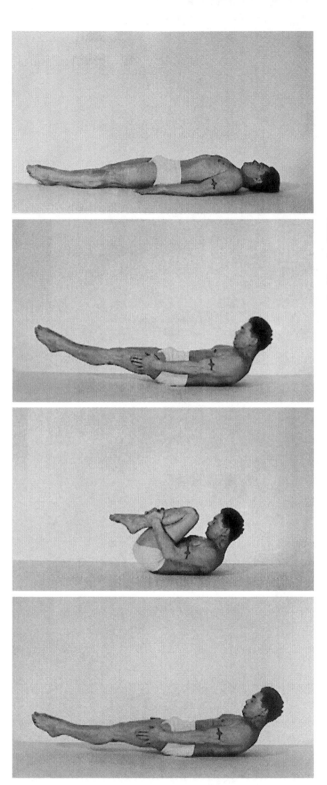

# The Double Leg Stretch

**Pose 1**    (a) Take position illustrated

              (b) Rest entire body on mat or floor

              (c) Legs (close together) straight forward

              (d) Knees locked

              (e) Toes (pointed) forward and downward

              (f) Arms stretched straight forward beside body

              (g) Palms down

**Pose 2**    (a) INHALE SLOWLY

              (b) Head up

              (c) Chin to chest

              (d) Arms stretched straight forward and

              (e) Pressed firmly against thighs

              (f) Heels raised about 2" off mat or floor

              (g) Palms inward

**Pose 3**    (a) EXHALE SLOWLY

              (b) "Draw" both legs upward and forward and with

              (c) Locked wrists hold them firmly in "doubled-up" position
                   as indicated

              (d) "Pull" legs toward you and press them firmly against chest

**Pose 4**    (a) INHALE SLOWLY

**NOTE**    Repeat the foregoing exercise six (6) times. Later to twelve (12).

**CAUTIONS**    Pose 2 – Head pressed firmly against chest. Abdomen in. Heels raised
                  about 2" off mat or floor.

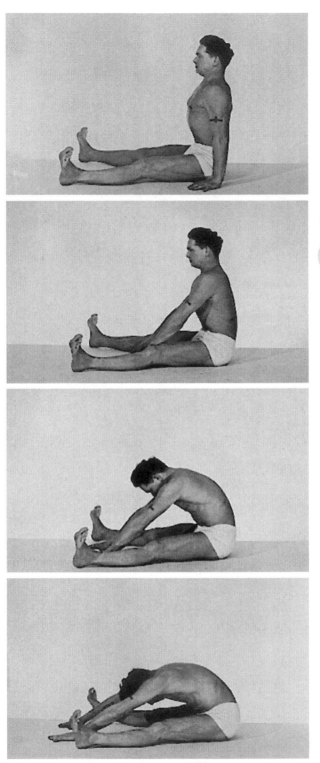

**8** The Spine Stretch

**Pose 1**    (a) Take position illustrated

             (b) Spread legs as wide apart as possible

             (c) "Draw" toes (pointed) upward and backward

**Pose 2**    (a) Rest palms flat on mat or floor, then with

             (b) Outstretched arms, palms flat on mat or floor

             (c) Chin touching chest

             (d) Begin reaching forward with three (3) successive "sliding" motion-stretching movements as far forward as possible until you assume position as illustrated in Poses 3 and 4

*NOTE*    Repeat the foregoing exercise three (3) times, trying with each repetition to reach farther and farther forward as indicated.

*CAUTIONS*    Pose 4 – Continue EXHALING SLOWLY, abdomen "drawn" in, chin pressed firmly against chest.

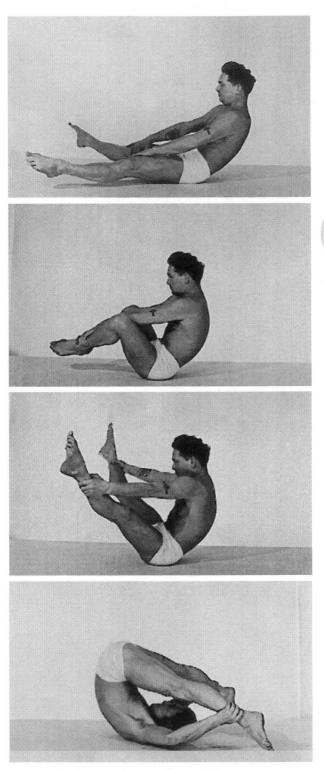

**Rocker With
Open Legs**

**Pose 1**    (a) Take position illustrated

**Pose 2**    (a) Bend knees
          (b) INHALE SLOWLY

**Pose 3**    (a) Grasp ankles firmly
          (b) Toes (pointed) forward and downward (knees locked)
          (c) Spread legs upward and outward as far as possible
          (d) Keep abdomen "drawn" in as far as possible with
          (e) Chin touching chest

**Pose 4**    (a) EXHALE SLOWLY
          (b) "Roll" over backward trying to touch mat or floor with toes

**NOTE**    Repeat the foregoing "rocking" exercise backward and forward six (6) times.

**CAUTIONS**    Pose 3 – Arms and legs rigid (elbows and knees locked). "Pivot" on base of spine, "rocking" backward to Pose 4 – position, then "rock" forward, pressing head firmly against chest, at the same time pressing arms firmly forward against legs until you reach Pose 3 and try to balance yourself in that position.

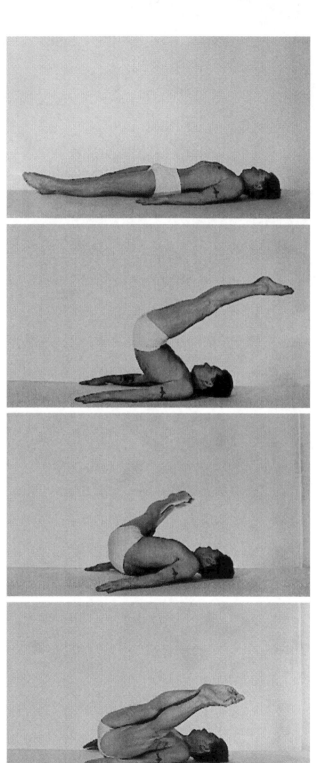

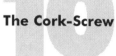

**Pose 1**    (a) Take position illustrated
            (b) Entire spine must rest on floor or mat
            (c) Arms straight forward touching body
            (d) Palms down

**Pose 2**    (a) INHALE SLOWLY
            (b) Raise legs (close together) "rolling" upward until
            (c) Body rests on shoulders, arms and head
            (d) Knees locked
            (e) Toes (pointed) forward and downward

**Pose 3**    (a) EXHALE SLOWLY
            (b) Lower both legs (close together) but not touching mat or floor
            (c) Knees locked
            (d) Toes (pointed) forward and downward
            (e) Twist trunk "corkscrew" fashion until
            (f) Body is partially lowered on right side to mat or floor

**Pose 4**    (a) INHALE SLOWLY
            (b) Make a complete right-to-left circle upward as far as possible
            (c) Return to Pose 2 position

**Pose 3**    (a) EXHALE SLOWLY
            (b) Lower both legs (close together) but not touching mat or floor
            (c) Knees locked
            (d) Toes (pointed) forward and downward
            (e) Twist trunk "corkscrew" fashion until
            (f) Body is partially lowered on left side to mat or floor

**Pose 4**    (a) INHALE SLOWLY
            (b) Make a complete left-to-right circle upward as far as possible
            (c) Return to Pose 2 position

**NOTE**    Repeat the foregoing exercise three (3) times each.

**CAUTIONS**    Pose 3 – While "circling" keep both shoulders pressed to mat or floor.
                  Arms straight.
            Pose 4 – While "circling" keep both shoulders pressed to mat or floor.
                  Arms straight.

**REMARKS**    This exercise strengthens neck and shoulders and is an internal and
            spinal massage.

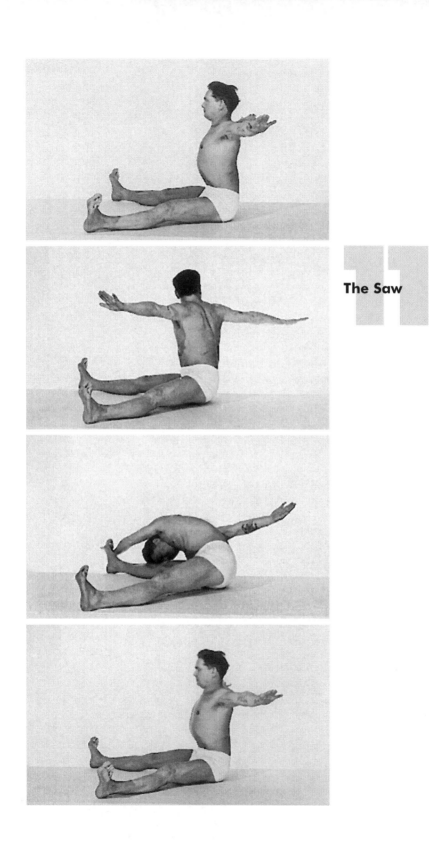

**Pose 1**    (a) Take position as illustrated
              (b) Spread legs as wide apart as possible
              (c) Head up
              (d) Chin "drawn" in
              (e) Chest out
              (f) Abdomen "drawn" in
              (g) Arms (shoulder-high) pressed backward until shoulder blades lock
              (h) INHALE SLOWLY

**Pose 2**    (a) Twist body (from trunk only) to right as far as possible

**Pose 3**    (a) Bend forward and downward as far as possible until
              (b) Left hand crosses and rests diagonally and centrally on right foot
              (c) EXHALE SLOWLY while
              (d) Stretching body forward in three (3) successive sliding-reaching "saw-like" motions as far as possible

**Pose 4**    (a) Resume position illustrated in this pose
              (b) INHALE SLOWLY

**Pose 2**    (a) Twist body (from trunk only) to left as far as possible

**Pose 3**    (a) Bend forward and downward as far as possible until right hand crosses and rests diagonally and centrally on left foot
              (b) EXHALE SLOWLY while
              (c) Stretching body forward in three (3) successive sliding-reaching "saw-like" motions as far as possible.

*NOTE*    Repeat the foregoing exercise three (3) times each.

*CAUTIONS*    Pose 2 – Twist body before bending forward as in Pose 3.
                Pose 3 – Lift raised arm backward and upward as high as possible as indicated in this pose.

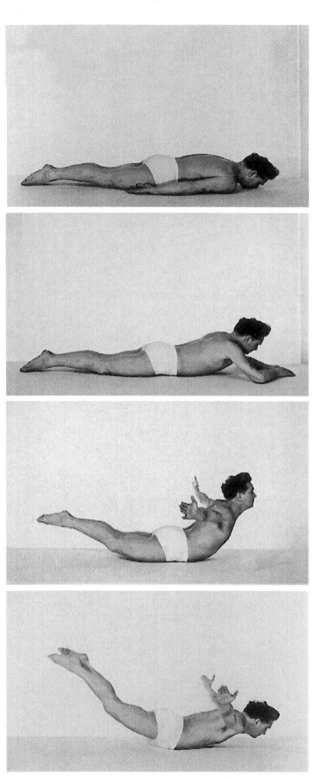

## The Swan-Dive

**Pose 1**    Take position illustrated

**Pose 2**    Take position illustrated

**Pose 3**
(a) INHALE SLOWLY
(b) Head raised upward and backward as far as possible
(c) Chest raised high from mat or floor
(d) Raise arms upward and sideward in line with locked shoulders
(e) Turn palms upward (right to left)
(f) Legs (close together) stretched and raised off mat or floor
(g) Toes (pointed) forward and downward (knees locked)
(h) Body rigid
(i) Back locked

**Pose 4**
(a) EXHALE SLOWLY as you "rock" forward
(b) INHALE SLOWLY as you "rock" upward

*NOTE*    Repeat the foregoing "rocking" exercise six (6) times.

*CAUTIONS*    Pose 3 – Keep back locked, legs off mat or floor, head back, arms rigid, shoulders locked.

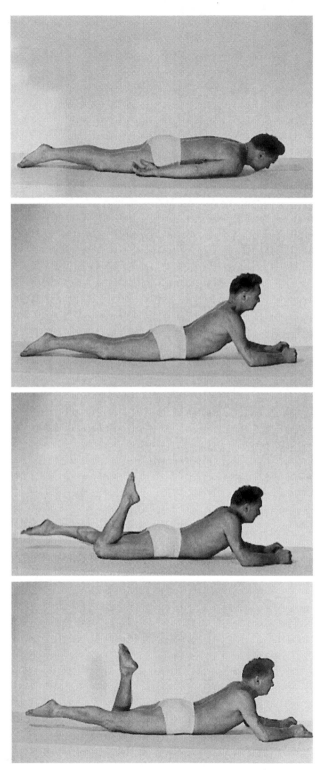

# The One Leg Kick

**Pose 1**    (a) Take position illustrated
              (b) Lie flat with head resting on arms
              (c) Stretch legs (close together) straight backward
              (d) Knees locked
              (e) Toes (pointed) forward and downward

**Pose 2**    (a) Lie on abdomen
              (b) Head up
              (c) Raise chest above mat or floor
              (d) Stretch arms forward to right angle position
              (e) Rest clenched fists on mat or floor
              (f) Stretch legs (close together) straight backward
              (g) Keep knees locked
              (h) Toes (pointed) forward and downward

**Pose 3**    (a) INHALE SLOWLY and
              (b) Raise legs about 2" above mat or floor
              (c) Try to snap-kick heel of right leg to buttocks

**Pose 4**    (a) EXHALE SLOWLY while
              (b) Stretching right leg backward and with
              (c) Heel of left leg
              (d) Try to snap-kick heel of left leg to buttocks

**NOTE**    Repeat the foregoing exercise six (6) times-right and left.

**CAUTIONS**    Pose 2 – Head up. Chest above mat or floor.
                  Pose 3 – Keep toes (pointed) above mat or floor.

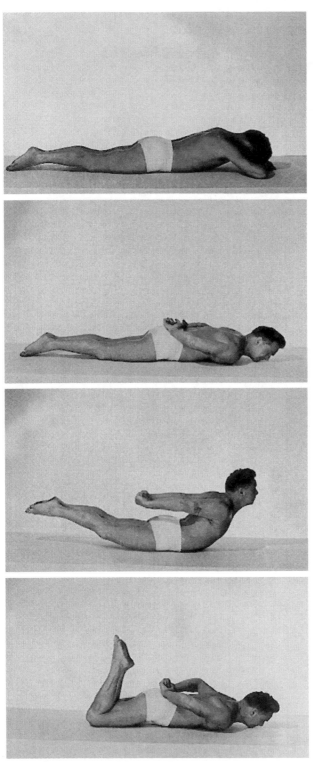

## The Double Kick

**Pose 1**    (a) Take position illustrated

(b) Arms stretched backward

(c) Firmly pressed to sides of body

(d) Fists clenched

(e) Face down and

(f) Chin touching mat or floor

(g) Toes (pointed) forward and downward

(h) Knees locked

**Pose 2**    (a) Rest chin on mat or floor

(b) Fold arms backward

(c) Grasp fingers of left hand with right hand

(d) Stretch legs (close together) straight backward

(e) Knees locked

(f) Toes (pointed) backward and downward and

(g) Raised about 1" above mat or floor

**Pose 3**    (a) Raise legs forward to right angle position

**Pose 4**    (a) INHALE SLOWLY

(b) Thrust chest out with head thrown back as far as possible and at the same time

(c) Raise arms (locked) from body

(d) Stretch backward (tensed) as far as possible, then

(e) Snap-kick legs (tensed) straight backward and

(f) Raised as high as possible from mat or floor

**NOTE**    Repeat foregoing exercise five (5) times.

**CAUTIONS**    Pose 4 – Keep head up as high as possible. Keep arms stretched backward as far as possible without touching body.

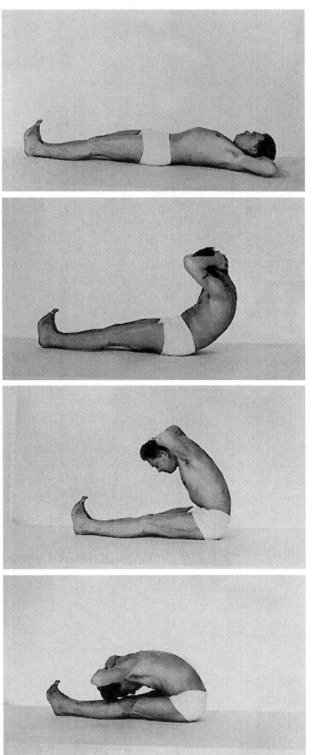

**Pose 1**    (a) Take position illustrated

            (b) INHALE SLOWLY

            (c) Clasp hands (fingers firmly interlocked) behind head

            (d) Toes (pointed) up and backward

**Pose 2**    (a) Bend head forward, chin touching chest

            (b) Abdomen "drawn" in

            (c) Toes (pointed) upward

            (d) Spine "bowed" forward off mat or floor

**Pose 3**    (a) EXHALE SLOWLY

            (b) Tense and press legs firmly downward against mat or floor

            (c) Slowly raise body upward and forward to position as indicated

            (d) Toes (pointed) upward

**Pose 4**    (a) EXHALE SLOWLY

            (b) Bend body forward until head and knees meet, if possible, as illustrated

            (c) Keep elbows straight backward until shoulder blades lock

            (d) INHALE SLOWLY while

            (e) Returning to Pose 3 position

            (f) EXHALE SLOWLY while

            (g) Returning to Poses 2 and 1 positions

*NOTE*    Repeat the foregoing exercise three (3) times.

*CAUTIONS*    Pose 1 – Keep toes (pointed) upward.

              Pose 2 – Keep legs pressed firmly to mat or floor (if necessary, placing cushion on feet).

              Pose 4 – Elbows straight backward until shoulder blades lock.

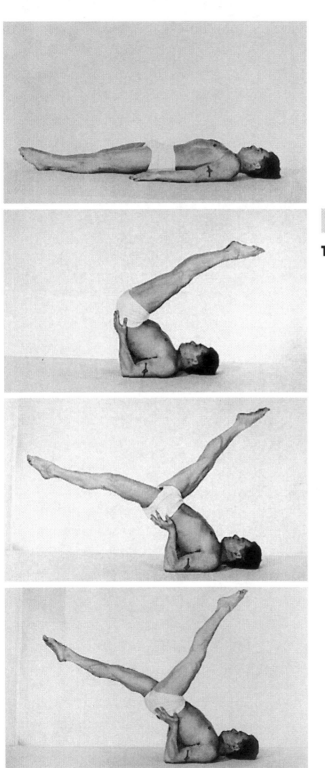

**Pose 1**    (a) Take position illustrated

**Pose 2**    (a) Bring legs upward until
             (b) Your body rests on head, shoulders, upper arms, neck and elbows, then with
             (c) "Cupped" hands supporting hips
             (d) INHALE SLOWLY

**Pose 3**    (a) "Split" legs scissors-like (left leg backward; right leg forward)
             (b) Legs stretched (knees locked)
             (c) Toes (pointed) forward and downward

**Pose 4**    (a) EXHALE SLOWLY
             (b) Alternate "split" legs scissors-like (right leg backward; left leg forward)

**NOTE**    Repeat the foregoing scissors-like exercise six (6) times.

**CAUTIONS**    Pose 2 – Keep body rigid, move legs only, knees locked, toes (pointed) forward and downward. Try gradually to execute "split" so that toes of forward leg, in alternating movements, are beyond your vision; and backward leg, in alternating movements, likewise.

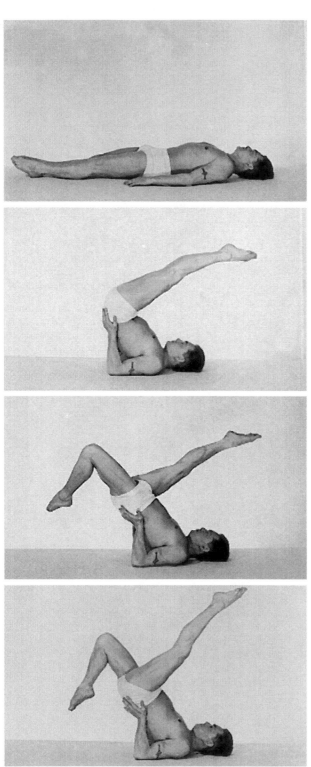

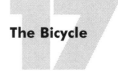

**The Bicycle**

**Pose 1**    (a) Take position illustrated

**Pose 2**    (a) Raise body on arms, elbows, shoulders, neck, and head
          (b) INHALE SLOWLY
          (c) "Split" legs (Pose 3)

**Pose 3**    (a) Bend right knee downward and backward and try to
             "kick" yourself
          (b) EXHALE SLOWLY

**Pose 4**    (a) "Pull" right leg straight backward
          (b) INHALE SLOWLY
          (c) Bend left knee downward and backward and try to
             "kick" yourself

*NOTE*    Repeat the foregoing "kicking" exercise five (5) times with each leg.

*CAUTIONS*    Pose 3 – Be sure to assume position as nearly as possible to that illustrated in this pose. Stretch each leg alternately forward beyond your vision with knee locked, toes (pointed) forward and downward.

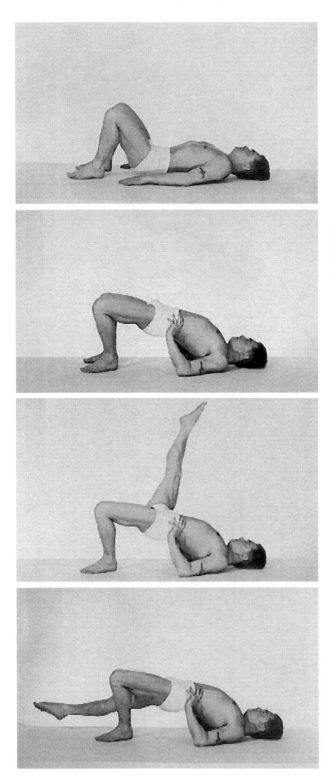

**Pose 1**    (a) Take position illustrated

**Pose 2**    (a) Raise body on upper arms, elbows, shoulders, neck, head, with both feet flat on mat or floor
        (b) Grasp waist firmly with both hands as illustrated

**Pose 3**    (a) INHALE SLOWLY
        (b) Raise right leg forward and upward to upright position
        (c) Toes (pointed) forward and downward

**Pose 4**    (a) EXHALE SLOWLY
        (b) Lower right leg forward and downward without bending knee and with knee locked
        (c) Thrust chest upward and outward as far as possible as illustrated in this pose

**Pose 3**    (a) INHALE SLOWLY
        (b) Raise left leg forward and upward to upright position
        (c) Toes (pointed) forward and downward

**Pose 4**    (a) EXHALE SLOWLY
        (b) Lower left leg forward and downward without bending knee and with knee locked
        (c) Thrust chest upward and outward as far as possible as illustrated in this pose

*NOTE*    Repeat left leg and right leg movements three (3) times.

*CAUTIONS*    Pose 3 – Toes pointed, knee locked right leg. Press foot firmly downward on mat or floor as each leg is lowered and chest thrust out.

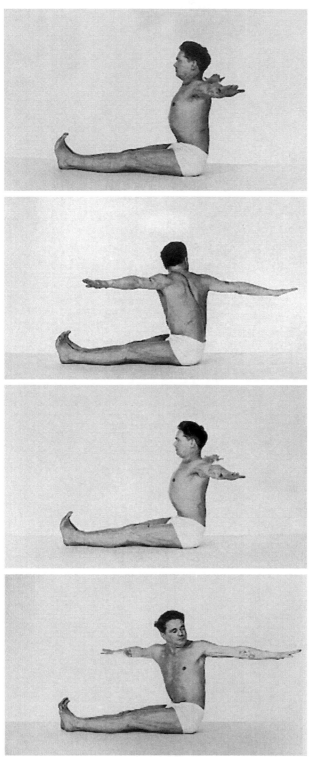

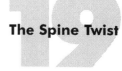

**The Spine Twist**

**Pose 1**    (a) Take position illustrated
         (b) INHALE SLOWLY
         (c) Sit perfectly upright in right angle position
         (d) Chest out
         (e) Abdomen "drawn" in
         (f) Head up
         (g) Arms (shoulder-wide, palms down) stretched backward until shoulder blades lock
         (h) Legs (close together) resting full length on mat or floor
         (i) Toes (pointed) upward and backward

**Pose 2**    (a) Keeping arms and legs absolutely rigid
         (b) EXHALE SLOWLY while
         (c) Twisting body and turning head to right as far as possible, then with two (2) further supreme mental and physical efforts, strive to better your original first attempt
         (d) INHALE SLOWLY while
         (e) Returning to position in

**Pose 3**    (a) Illustration

**Pose 4**    (a) EXHALE SLOWLY while
         (b) Twisting body and turning head to left as far as possible, then with two (2) further supreme mental and physical efforts, strive to better your original first attempt
         (c) INHALE SLOWLY while
         (d) Returning to position in

**Pose 3**    (a) Illustration

**NOTE**    Repeat the foregoing exercise three (3) times left and three (3) times right, trying with each repetition to reach farther and farther backward.

**CAUTIONS**    Pose 1 – Keep arms and legs absolutely rigid. Shoulder blades locked. Twist body from spine only. Try to touch chin alternately to right and left shoulder.

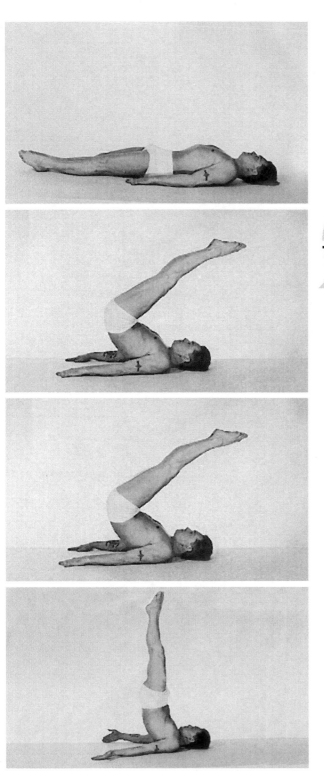

**Pose 1**    (a) Take position illustrated

            (b) Rest entire spine on mat or floor

**Pose 2**    (a) Stretch arms sidewise

            (b) Both legs (close together) raised upward to right angle position

            (c) Knees locked

            (d) Toes (pointed) forward and downward

            (e) INHALE SLOWLY

**Pose 3**    (a) Press arms firmly downward against mat or floor

            (b) With knees locked "roll" body over until

            (c) Spine is raised off mat or floor (about 5")

**Pose 4**    (a) "Kick" legs in snappy "jack-knife" fashion straight upward until

            (b) Entire body rests on head, neck, shoulders, arms

            (c) EXHALE SLOWLY

            (d) Return to Pose 3 position

            (e) INHALE SLOWLY and then

            (f) Return to Pose 2 position

            (g) EXHALE SLOWLY

*NOTE*    Repeat the foregoing exercise three (3) times.

*CAUTIONS*    Pose 2 – Keep legs in right angle position, knees locked, toes pointed.
                  Pose 3 – Hold Pose 3 position for mental count of 2.
                  Pose 4 – Hold Pose 4 position for mental count of 2.

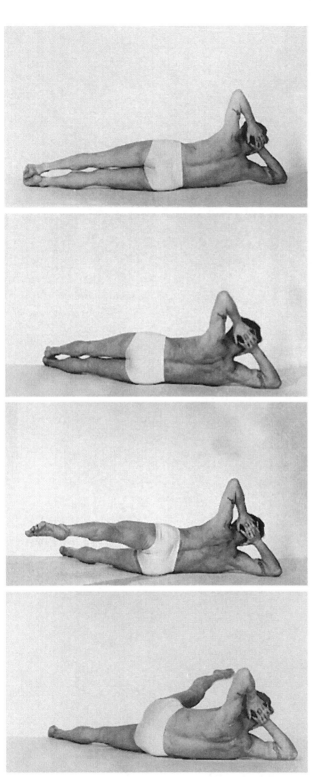

21
The Side Kick

**Pose 1**    (a) Take position illustrated

                (b) Lock hands behind head

                (c) Head up

                (d) Eyes straight forward

                (e) Arms straight in line with shoulders

                (f) Lie full length right side on mat or floor

**Pose 2**    (a) Bring legs (close together) forward about 2 feet

                (a) INHALE SLOWLY

                (b) "Swing" left leg forward as far as possible to you

                (c) Return left leg about 1 foot backward and

                (d) "Swing" left leg forward to you again and attempt to better your first trial

**Pose 3**    (a) INHALE SLOWLY, turn around and

                (b) "Swing" right leg forward as far as possible to you

                (c) Return right leg about 1 foot backward and

                (d) "Swing" right leg forward to you again and attempt to better your first trial

**Pose 4**    (a) EXHALE SLOWLY

                (b) "Swing" right leg backward as far as possible

                (c) Return right leg about 1 foot forward and

                (d) "Swing" right leg backward again and attempt to better your first trial

**NOTE**    Repeat the foregoing exercise three (3) times, left and right.

**CAUTIONS**    Pose 3 – Head up, elbows back. Keep entire body rigid. Move "free" leg only. Keep other leg in straight line pressed against mat or floor.

                    Pose 4 – Maintain balance lying on side of body.

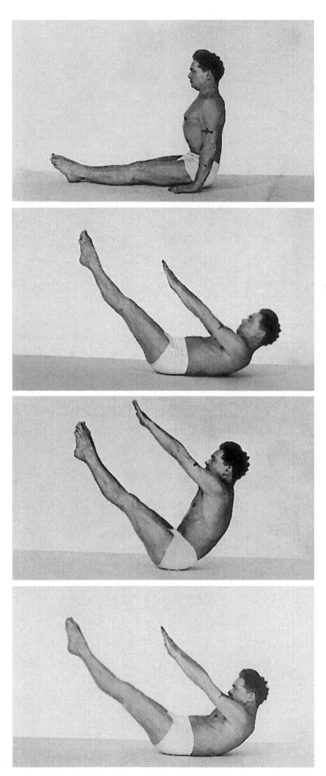

**Pose 1**    (a) Take position illustrated
        (b) Head up
        (c) Legs (close together)
        (d) Knees locked
        (e) Toes (pointed) forward and downward
        (f) Arms at right angle position beside body
        (g) Hands pointed straight forward

**Pose 2**    (a) Bend head forward
        (b) Chin to chest
        (c) Press abdomen in
        (d) "Roll" backward on spine until
        (e) Legs are raised upward to indicated angle

**Pose 3**    (a) INHALE SLOWLY
        (b) Raise arms in parallel line with legs as indicated

**Pose 4**    (a) "Roll" forward and upward
        (b) "Pivot" on rump keeping
        (c) Raised arms in line with raised legs as indicated (parallel)
        (d) EXHALE SLOWLY and
        (e) Return to Pose 2 position and
        (f) INHALE SLOWLY

***NOTE***    Repeat the foregoing exercise three (3) times.

***CAUTIONS***    Pose 3 – Arms and legs must be kept in straight parallel lines.
                Keep back well rounded. Chest pressed in.

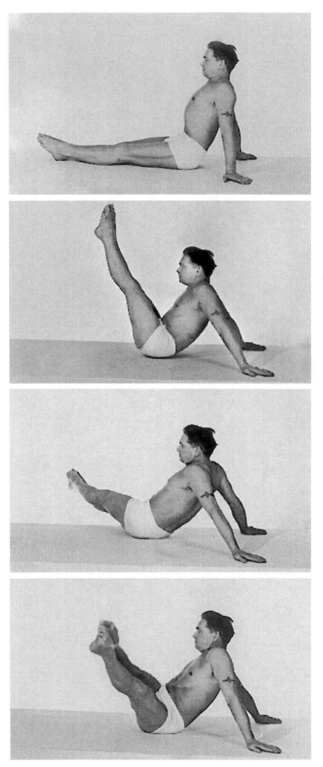

# The Hip Twist With Stretched Arms

**Pose 1**    (a) Take position illustrated

           (b) Put arms in right angle position

           (c) Firmly pressed to mat or floor with

           (d) Palms of hands in backward position

           (e) Keep legs (close together) straight forward

           (f) Keep toes (pointed) forward and downward

**Pose 2**    (a) INHALE SLOWLY

           (b) Swing legs (close together)

           (c) Knees locked

           (d) Toes (pointed) forward and downward

           (e) As high as possible

**Pose 3**    (a) EXHALE SLOWLY on downward

           (b) "Swing" without legs touching mat or floor

**Pose 4**    (a) INHALE SLOWLY

           (b) "Swing" legs upward as high as possible in righthand circle

           (c) EXHALE SLOWLY and start to

           (d) "Swing" legs downward in lefthand circle as far as possible

           (e) Without legs touching mat or floor

**NOTE**    Repeat the foregoing exercise three (3) times in succession – three (3) times for left circle, and three (3) times for righthand circle leg "swing" movements.

**CAUTIONS**    Pose 1 – Press chest inward as far as possible.

                Pose 2 – Chin down.

                Pose 4 – When "circling" upward "swing" legs as high and as close to head as possible. Be sure only legs and hips are moved.

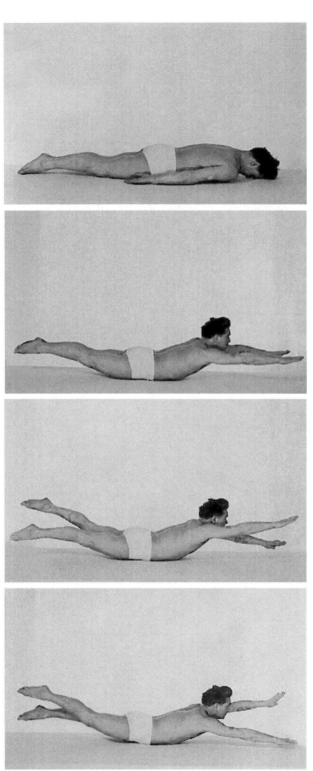

**Pose 1**    (a) Take position illustrated
**and**       (b) Arms stretched forward
**Pose 2**    (c) Palms down
           (d) Head upward and backward as far as possible
           (e) Chest raised off mat or floor
           (f) Toes (pointed) forward and downward
           (g) Knees locked
           (h) INHALE and EXHALE normally while performing the simultaneous, alternating, compound motions in the following movements, counting mentally from 1 to 10, beginning with right arm movement

**Pose 3**    (a) Left leg and right arm raised upward as far as possible and simultaneously reverse to

**Pose 4**    (a) Right leg and left arm position and follow instructions under (h) in 2 above

**NOTE**    Repeat the foregoing exercise as indicated in the preceding instructions.

**CAUTIONS**    Pose 3 – Left leg and right arm raised as high as possible in upward movements. Left leg and right arm must not touch mat or floor in downward movements. Right leg and left arm raised as high as possible in upward movements. Right leg and left arm must not touch mat or floor in downward movements. Keep body rigid. Move arms and legs only.

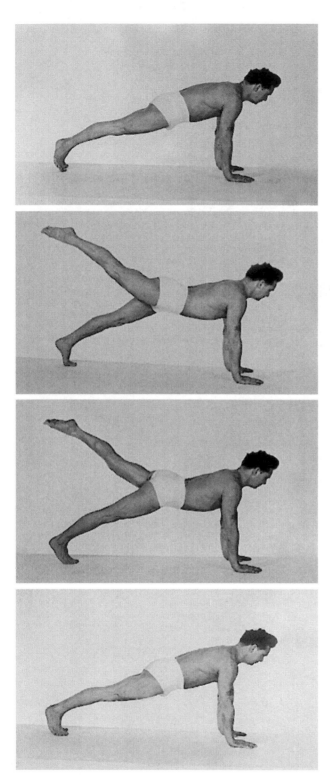

**Pose 1**    (a) Take position illustrated

       (b) Arms (shoulder-wide) in right angle position

       (c) Hands at right angles

       (d) Head in straight line with body

       (e) Legs close together

       (f) Toes (pointed) downward

       (g) Heels close together

       (h) Knees locked

**Pose 2**    (a) INHALE SLOWLY

       (b) Raise right leg upward and backward as high as possible

       (c) EXHALE SLOWLY

       (d) Lower right leg to Pose 1 position

**Pose 3**    (a) INHALE SLOWLY

       (b) Raise left leg upward and backward as high as possible

       (c) EXHALE SLOWLY

       (d) Lower left leg to Pose 1 position

*NOTE*    Repeat the foregoing exercise three (3) times, right and left.

*CAUTIONS*    Pose 1 – Arms must be shoulder-wide in right angle position.
       Pose 2 – Move legs only, knees locked.
       Pose 3 – Move legs only, knees locked.

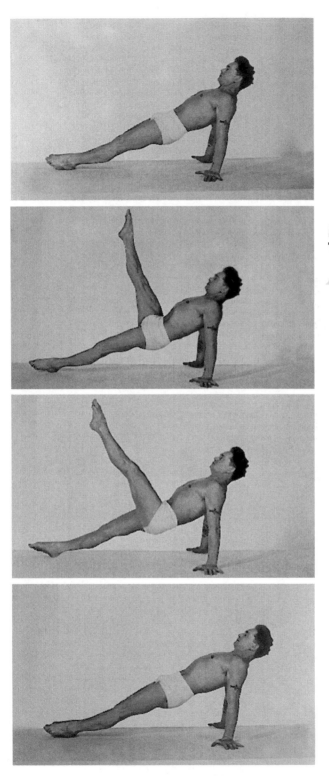

**Pose 1**    (a) Take position illustrated

(b) Arms (shoulder-wide) in right angle position

(c) Hands at right angles

(d) Head in straight line with body

(e) Legs close together

(f) Toes pointed downward

(g) Heels close together

(h) Knees locked

**Pose 2**    (a) INHALE SLOWLY

(b) Raise right leg upward and backward as high as possible

(c) EXHALE SLOWLY

(d) Lower right leg to Pose 1 position

**Pose 3**    (a) INHALE SLOWLY

(b) Raise left leg upward and backward as high as possible

(c) EXHALE SLOWLY

(d) Lower left leg to Pose 1 position

*NOTE*    Repeat the foregoing leg exercise three (3) times, right and left.

*CAUTIONS*    Pose 1 – Arms must be shoulder-wide in right angle position.
Pose 2 – Move legs only, knees locked.
Pose 3 – Move legs only, knees locked.

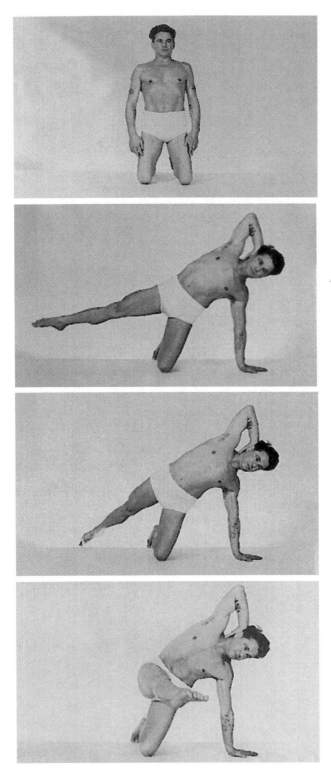

## The Side Kick Kneeling

## 27

**Pose 1**    (a) Take position illustrated

**Pose 2**    (a) Kneel on left knee and
        (b) Support body on left arm, then
        (c) Stretch right leg (knee locked) out sidewise in straight line
            with body
        (d) Toes (pointed) forward and downward, then
        (e) Bring right arm backward with hand supporting head, elbow
            back as far as possible, then

**Pose 3**    (a) INHALE QUICKLY while
        (b) "Swinging" right leg backward forcibly as far as possible, then

**Pose 4**    (a) EXHALE QUICKLY while
        (b) "Swinging" right leg forward forcibly as far as possible

**Pose 2**    (a) Kneel on right knee and
        (b) Support body on right arm, then
        (c) Stretch left leg (knee locked) out sidewise in straight line
            with body with
        (d) Toes (pointed) forward and downward, then
        (e) Bring left arm and elbow backward as far as possible with
            hand supporting head, then

**Pose 3**    (a) INHALE QUICKLY while
        (b) "Swinging" left leg backward forcibly as far as possible, then

**Pose 4**    (a) EXHALE QUICKLY while
        (b) "Swinging" left leg backward forcibly as far as possible

*NOTE*    Repeat the foregoing exercise four times with each leg.

*CAUTIONS*    Pose 2 – Keep head up, elbow back, chest out and abdomen in.
            Keep body rigid; move legs only. INHALE QUICKLY when
            swinging legs forcibly forward. EXHALE QUICKLY when
            swinging legs forcibly backward.

*REMARKS*    Concentrating on waistline and hips, also exercise for balance and
          coordination.

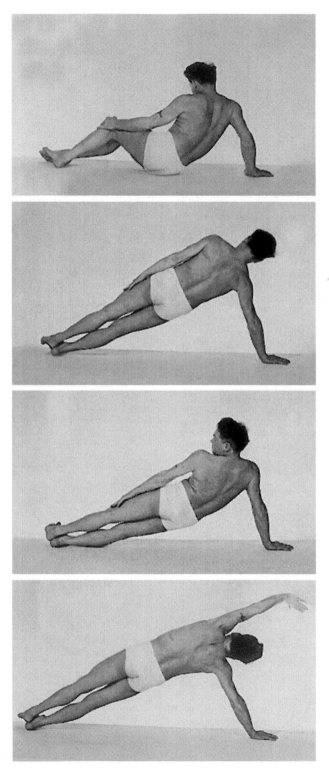

**The Side Bend**

## 28

**Pose 1**    (a) Take position illustrated

**Pose 2**    (a) Keep right arm in line with right shoulder
           (b) Left arm flat against body
           (c) Head up
           (d) Chin "drawn" in
           (e) Eyes straight forward
           (f) INHALE SLOWLY

**Pose 3**    (a) Turn head left and try to rest chin on left shoulder
           (b) Lower body until right calf touches mat or floor
           (c) EXHALE SLOWLY
           (d) Return to Pose 2 position
           (e) INHALE SLOWLY

**Pose 2**    (a) Keep left arm in line with left shoulder
           (b) Right arm flat against body
           (c) Head up
           (d) Chin "drawn" in
           (e) Eyes straight forward
           (f) INHALE SLOWLY

**Pose 3**    (a) Turn head right and try to rest chin on right shoulder
           (b) Lower body until left calf touches mat or floor
           (c) EXHALE SLOWLY
           (d) Return to Pose 2 position
           (e) INHALE SLOWLY

**NOTE**    Repeat the foregoing exercise three (3) times, right and left.

**CAUTIONS**    Pose 2 – Keep body rigid, head up, chest out, abdomen "drawn" in.
           Pose 3 – Only left and right calf respectively should touch mat
                 when lowered.

**REMARKS**    This exercise concentrates on arm, shoulder and wrist muscles, stretches
           hip and waistline, and develops balance and coordination. In a month,
           change from Pose 2 position to Pose 4.

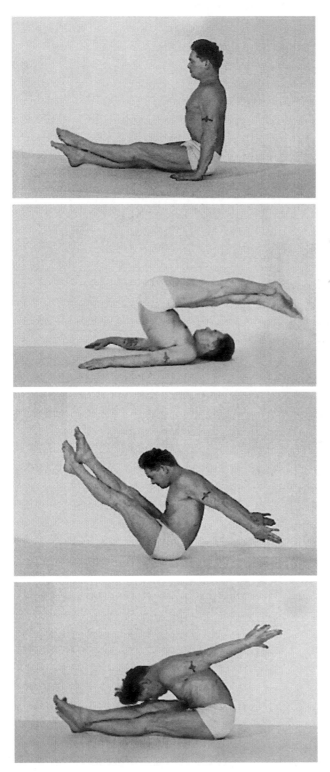

**Pose 1**   (a) Take position illustrated

(b) INHALE SLOWLY

(c) Sit up straight in right angle position

(d) Head up

(e) Abdomen "drawn" in

(f) Cross left leg over right leg

(g) Arms pressed against body

(h) Hands pointed forward and pressed against mat or floor

**Pose 2**   (a) EXHALE SLOWLY while

(b) "Rolling" backward as far as possible and while in this position

(c) Cross right leg over left leg and

**Pose 3**   (a) INHALE SLOWLY while

(b) "Rolling" forward and

(c) "Swing" arms backward as far as possible

**Pose 4**   (a) EXHALE SLOWLY while bringing both

(b) Legs to mat or floor with

(c) Head touching knees with

(d) Arms (palms up) raised backward as far as possible and upward and

(e) Return to Pose 2 position

**NOTE**   Repeat the foregoing exercise six (6) times, first starting with right leg crossed over left leg and then crossing left leg over right leg alternately.

**CAUTIONS**   Pose 2 – Keep arms and shoulders pressed firmly against mat or floor. Reverse legs while in "overhead" position when returning to Pose 3 position.
Pose 4 – Try to touch head to knees. Keep arms (palms up) stretched straight backward and upward as far as possible.

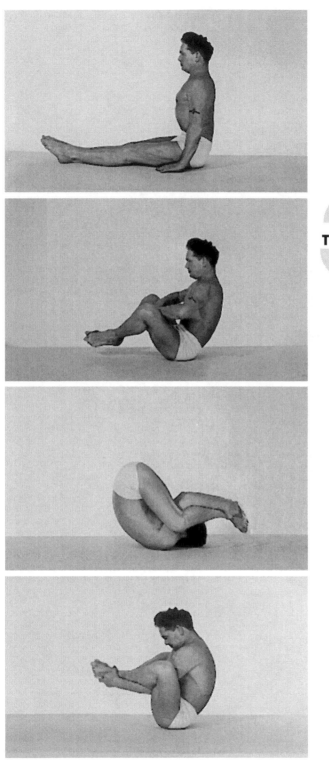

**Pose 1**    (a) Take position illustrated

**Pose 2**    (a) INHALE SLOWLY
           (b) Bend head forward to chest
           (c) Abdomen pressed in
           (d) Legs apart "spread-eagle" fashion
           (e) Soles and heels together, pointed inward

**Pose 3**    (a) EXHALE SLOWLY
           (b) Twine both arms "grape-vine" fashion under both legs
           (c) Passing left arm under and over left leg
           (d) Grasping left instep in locked grip
           (e) Passing right arm under and over right leg
           (f) Grasping right instep in locked grip
           (g) Press soles and heels firmly close together, pointed inward

**Pose 4**    (a) INHALE SLOWLY while
           (b) "Rolling" backward as far as possible
           (c) EXHALE SLOWLY
           (d) Return to Pose 3 position
           (e) "Clap" (hand-fashion) soles and heels together, twice

**NOTE**    Repeat the foregoing exercise six (6) times.

**CAUTIONS**    Pose 2 – Bend body forward. Press chest in. Tilt body backward to raise legs off mat or floor.
           Pose 3 – "Pivot" body on rump in "rolling" backward and forward. You INHALE while "rolling" backward.
           Pose 4 – Press head firmly to mat or floor in "rolling" upward. You EXHALE while "rolling" upward.

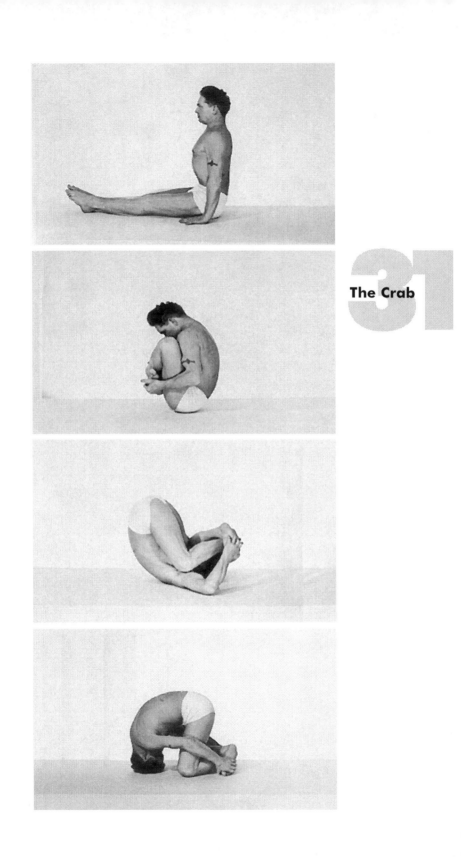

**Pose 1**    (a) Take position illustrated
           (b) INHALE SLOWLY

**Pose 2**    (a) EXHALE SLOWLY
           (b) Cross legs Indian-fashion
           (c) Head bent forward
           (d) Chin to chest
           (e) Abdomen pressed in
           (f) Grasp both feet firmly
           (g) Right hand grasping left foot
           (h) Left hand grasping right foot
           (i) "Pull" both knees toward shoulders as far as possible

**Pose 3**    (a) INHALE SLOWLY while
           (b) "Rolling" backward as far as possible
           (c) EXHALE SLOWLY while
           (d) "Rolling" upward until

**Pose 4**    (a) Head rests on mat or floor
           (b) INHALE SLOWLY until you return to Pose 3 position
           (c) EXHALE SLOWLY while again "rolling" upward until
           (d) Head rests on mat or floor as indicated in Pose 4

**NOTE**    Repeat the foregoing exercise six (6) times.

**CAUTIONS**    Pose 2 – Hold head as closely as possible to chest. Press abdomen in. "Round" back. "Pull" knees to shoulders as nearly as possible. "Pivot" on rump.

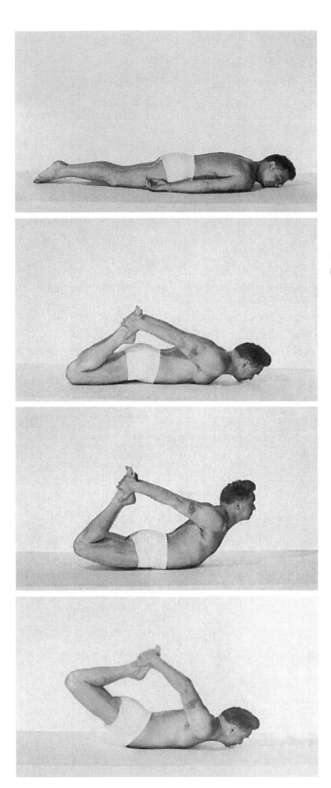

**Pose 1**     (a) Take position illustrated

                 (b) Rest body (face downward) on mat or floor

                 (c) Press arms to sides with palms upward

                 (d) Stretch legs (close together) backward

                 (e) Keep toes (pointed) forward and downward

**Pose 2**     (a) Bend legs forward toward head

                 (b) Grasp feet

**Pose 3**     (a) INHALE SLOWLY

                 (b) Thrust chest out with head thrown back as far as possible

                 (c) Stretch legs (close together) toward mat or floor

**Pose 4**     (a) Rock forward until chin touches mat or floor

                 (b) Rock backward as far as possible

                 (c) INHALE SLOWLY as you

                 (d) Rock forward and

                 (e) EXHALE SLOWLY as you

                 (f) Rock backward

**NOTE**     Repeat the foregoing exercise five (5) times.

**CAUTIONS**    Pose 2 – Keep head thrown back as far as possible.

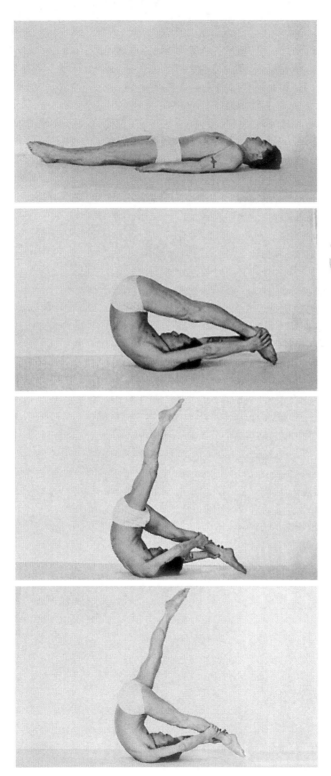

**Pose 1**    (a) Take position illustrated

        (b) Rest entire body on mat or floor

        (c) Legs (close together) straight forward

        (d) Ioes (pointed) forward and downward

        (e) Arms straight forward beside body

        (f) Palms down

**Pose 2**    (a) INHALE SLOWLY

        (b) "Roll" over until body rests on shoulders, arms and neck, and

        (c) Right toe touches mat or floor with

        (d) Right foot firmly grasped by both hands and

        (e) Left leg held straight upward as high as possible

**Pose 3**    (a) EXHALE SLOWLY

        (b) Release hold of hands on right foot and

        (c) Bring left leg downward until

        (d) Left toe touches mat or floor and

        (e) Grasp left foot firmly with both hands

        (f) Right leg held straight upward as high as possible

**NOTE**    Repeat the foregoing exercise six (6) times.

**CAUTIONS**    Pose 2 – Maintain balance on shoulders, arms and neck.
                Keep knees locked  Toes (pointed) forward and downward.

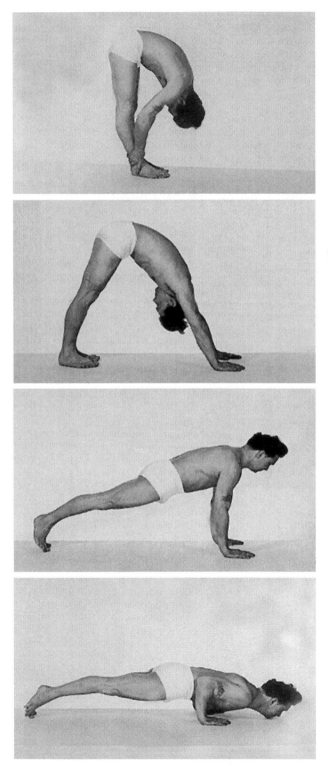

**Pose 1**    (a) Take position illustrated
                  (b) With arms (shoulder-wide) and palms extended
                  (c) Try to touch mat or floor

**Pose 2**    (a) Keep feet pressed firmly on mat or floor
                  (b) Proceed "to walk" forward on palms of hands
                  (c) Keep head downward and continue "walking" forward until

**Pose 3**    (a) You assume position illustrated in this pose
                  (b) Keep body rigid and in a straight line from head to heels
                  (c) Raise weight of body on toes and palms with
                  (d) Arms (shoulder-wide) and hands pointed straight forward
                  (e) Keep head in straight line with body

**Pose 4**    (a) Keep body rigid
                  (b) Back locked
                  (c) Bend arms (shoulder-wide) at elbows with
                  (d) Upper arms pressed firmly to body
                  (e) INHALE SLOWLY
                  (f) Lower body until chin touches mat or floor
                  (g) Stretch neck straight outward as far as possible
                  (h) Hips locked
                  (i) Abdomen "drawn" in
                  (j) Chest raised above mat or floor
                  (k) EXHALE SLOWLY
                  (l) Raise body slowly by
                  (m) Pressing hands firmly against mat or floor

**NOTE**    Repeat the foregoing exercise three (3) times.

**CAUTIONS**    Pose 3 – Keep shoulders in straight line with hands. Hips locked. Head in straight line with body. Keep body absolutely rigid. Move arms only (not body). Touch chin (not chest) to mat or floor.

*Return to Life*

Made in the USA
San Bernardino, CA
05 November 2019